Hair

How to Reduce the Effects of Male Pattern Baldness

By

ames Bernard Pinski, M.D., F.A.C.P., F.I.C.S

J.B. Media International
London • New York • La Jolla • Melbourne • Tokyo

ISBN 0-937043-02-8

ii

Table of Contents

Chapter   *Page*

One   Hair Restoration   1

Two   Self Image   9

Three   Hair Growth and Baldness   15

Four   Drugs, Hair and Treatment of Baldness   33

Five   Hair Pieces and Fiber Implants   37

Six   Surgical Hair Replacement   41

Seven   Scalp Reduction   71

Eight   Patient Selection and Hair   79

Nine   Procedure   83

Ten   Hair Transplant Questions   87

Chapter One
Hair Restoration

Hair loss is a common occurrence among men and less common among women, and although it may be distressing, in most cases it is a normal condition dictated by heredity. The exact hereditary pattern is not fully understood, although we do know that a tendency for baldness is passed on by both maternal and paternal ancestors. We call this occurrence in men and women, "pattern baldness."

Age is an important factor in typical male pattern baldness. Baldness in a man normally begins when he reaches his late teens or early twenties, and in a woman when she reaches her forties, and it progresses with age. Most men and some women lose hair at varying rates throughout their entire lives. For some this condition may only cause a gradual thinning of the hair. For others it rapidly produces baldness.

Male hormones, called androgens, are a significant factor in baldness. Baldness is not dependent on the quantity of androgens present, but merely on their presence. Androgens must be present to produce this type of hair loss. In men, androgen levels are normal. In women, ovarian function may fade, resulting in fewer female hormones being produced. Thus the male hormones normally present in small amounts, become, in effect, predominant. Research has shown that if a male is castrated in his early twenties, his production of male hormones practically ceases and baldness will be arrested. One might say that castration is a prevention for baldness, though not a logical approach to the problem.

Certain follicles (the factories which produce individual hairs) are pre-programmed to be sensitive to androgens. Apparently, follicles on the top and upper sides of the scalp are affected in this way and not on the lower sides and back of the scalp. Though the top of a man's head may become completely bald, he will not lose the hair on the lower sides of his scalp, neck, chest, armpits, or pubic area. It is from the non-balding or permanent areas of hair bearing scalp that autografts or hair replacement comes from.

The androgen named "testosterone" is chemically converted into another form called "dihydrotestosterone" by the action of the enzyme "alpha-reductase." It is the dihydrotestosterone that causes scalp follicles to produce progressively thinner and shorter hairs as they go through their growth cycles. This happens until thin or no hair grows in a given area.

In typical male pattern baldness, the hair at the front of the head may thin out first, creating a receding hairline, and the hair loss progresses gradually to the top of the head. Yet, the hair just above the ears and on the back of the head usually remains healthy and full, regardless of the dihydrotestosterone levels, producing the "monk's wreath" most common in male pattern baldness.

Of course not all groups of men experience the same type of baldness. Ethnic and racial groups show definite differences in their susceptibility to baldness. Hair loss is less common, for example, among black men than white. Then too, where there is a tendency for an ethnic group to experience baldness, inbreeding results in higher numbers of that group being bald. Illness, injury, certain drugs and a host of other things can cause baldness. Many times this type of baldness can be medically corrected or it may even correct itself over a period of time. Hair loss due to hereditarily-induced male pattern baldness is by far the most common form and will not correct itself, nor is hair likely to return short of medical or surgical procedures.

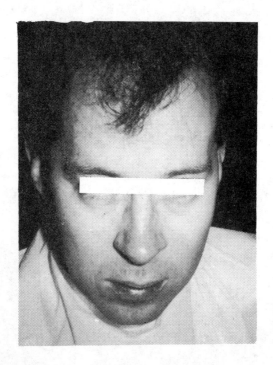

Before: This young man felt he was too young to have the degree of baldness that he displayed.

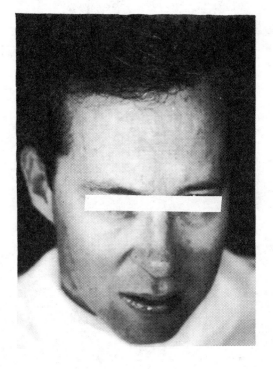

After: With hair transplantation, he enjoys a more youthful look and is pleased with his restored hairline.

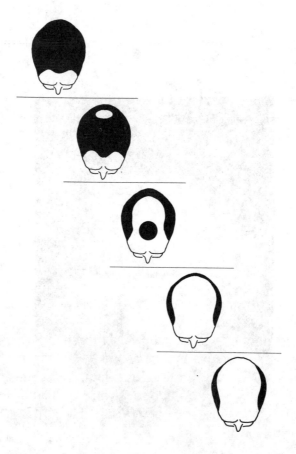

These drawings show the most common patterns of baldness.

By age 25, approximately twenty percent of men from European extraction will experience some degree of baldness. It is often seen as mild thinning over the front and crown of the head with a marked receding frontal hairline. By the time these men reach their 30s, the percentage of men experiencing baldness increases to about forty percent. At age 50 some form of baldness is present with half of all males. At age 60 the percentage climbs to seventy-five percent. Over a lifetime, more than two-thirds of all males of European descent exhibit some degree of baldness and half of those have little or no hair on the crown of their head with some degree of thinness along the sides.

Baldness normally begins in a predictable pattern. There are two types: 1) At the top back part of the head, spreading out across the crown, moving toward the front; 2) the front hairline, gradually receding backward to the crown and beyond. The second is the most common type.

In cases where baldness begins at the front hairline and recedes backward, there are two common patterns displayed. The hairline may thin or baldness result from the forehead to the upper back of the of head, or a tuft of hair may remain anchored in the center front. With the latter the appearance of baldness is lessened considerably. The actor, Clint Eastwood, has this type of baldness. It is called a "persistent frontal forelock". Eastwood's hairline and center tuft of hair have thinned somewhat, yet movie fans don't perceive him as bald. His appearance is simply that of a maturing man, although his hair stylist must do some creative things to keep up the appearance of having some hair. Each year he is losing more of his tuft. He appears to be an excellent candidate for a hair transplant.

Chapter Two
Self Image

How We Perceive Ourselves

At a point in our lives, while growing up, we form a mental image of ourselves. In time, we develop a full mental view of our face and body, an image of how we think others see us. When we look in a mirror, we identify with what we see and inwardly say, "That's me." Even without a mirror we have an idea of the image we project to the world.

As a man or a woman begins to bald, the appearance no longer matches the internal self-image developed over many years. This can be very disturbing, since we feel the same as before. When we see our reflection in the mirror, a different image confronts us. We may want to protest, "That isn't me."

The experience of going bald is part of the process of aging. At forty, most people feel much the same as they did at thirty or even twenty—more conservative, perhaps, certainly more mature. Yet within, the adult person remains as always. Confronted with baldness and aging, that person may begin to feel foreign to self and somewhat disoriented. This discomfort results in a desire to return "toward" the former appearance. It is not always possible, but in some areas one can correct the effects of aging.

It is not an unreasonable expectation to want to look the same as one feels. Most people at forty don't really expect to look twenty again, nor do many want to, but there is an increasing number of people who desire to look more youthful and want to increase their self-acceptance. In the case of baldness, many people miss the look of hair closely framing the face. Everyone has seen men, who have a dozen remaining hairs, make a low part at the side and carefully comb those strands across the top of the head. Even though those men know that the strands are not going to fool anyone, nevertheless they feel more comfortable with hair framing their faces. Others might think that they would look better bald, but they are happier with a look that conforms more closely to the facial self-image that they developed in their youth.

Undeniably, baldness does add age to a person's appearance, and it represents to men what wrinkles represent to women. (We refer not to the woman who is abnormally obsessed with looking age twenty forever, but to the mature woman who maintains that wrinkles don't properly represent what she knows herself to be.) Unfortunately, such attitudes are misconstrued as a form of vanity, which they are not. Vanity is a preoccupation with one's appearance and may represent a slight emotional instability. The desire to look better and project a more pleasing appearance is a normal human attitude and should be encouraged. If all the bald men in America could, through some form of magic instantly have a full head of hair, the consensus of opinion is that they would do just that. It is a natural preference. Although society tends to be youth-oriented, most members are not vainly preoccupied with perpetual youth. The way we look influences the way we behave and effects our confidence in our own abilities. Patients who consult with surgeons about correction of drooping eyelids remark that they are frequently asked by others if they are tired, when in fact they are not. They only appear that way.

Not to the same degree, but nevertheless a similar image applies to hair in our society. If you are bald there is a tendency for others to view you as older than you actually are. At least less youthful and less vibrant than if you had a full head of hair.

Following transplant surgery there is a change in an individual's appearance and confidence level. Before surgery, at times, a patient will look ill-groomed and retiring, less youthful and energetic. With a hair transplant there often comes a transformation. Many have a greater focus on life. Clearly there is a greatly enhanced appearance.

Of course, we can accept baldness. There are many who contend that it is unimportant. Yet, the media, especially television and movies place significant value on actors with hair. Men's magazines rarely display a man with thinning hair and almost never one who is bald. When the media displays a macho image of a man, he has a full head of hair. In this manner society associates having hair with a masculine look. It is also true with smooth, relatively unwrinkled skin, which somehow looks more tidy. It is not just hair that offers that well-groomed look. Eyelid correction, face-lifts, as well as hair restoration accomplish this more youthful appearance. Why else do you see so many older actors who look virile and alive, who have few wrinkles, a good head of hair and a youthful skin tone? Because that look has appeal.

When women were asked in several surveys whether they thought men looked better bald or with hair, a majority replied baldness did not influence their attraction to the opposite sex.

Yet, when shown photos of men with and without hair, those same women said repeatedly that the men with hair looked more attractive to them.

Many men may never admit it, and you may be saying, "Why make such an issue of hair replacement? It's just hair and little else." Maybe so, but entire industries have sprung up from man's desire to have a full, well-groomed head of hair. Try to convince these thriving companies that the focus is just hair. It is appearance, acceptance and satisfaction with for most individuals—not some imaginary desire.

Chapter Three
Hair Growth and Baldness

Normal Hair Growth

Hair seen on the outside of the skin is the upper part of the hair shaft. It is a complex weaving of lifeless protein produced by a hair root in a deep layer of scalp that is encased in a teardrop-shaped hair follicle which nourishes the root.

Hair has a normal cycle of growth. Its growing phase, called anagen, lasts for a variable number of years. Each follicle produces a hair during that time, which continues to grow at about a half inch per month.

The second phase is the catagen phase, during which hair is in a resting state for a brief period. Nutrition supplied by the follicle to the hair decreases during this time.

The third phase is call telogen and lasts for approximately three months. The follicle is present and healthy, but the hair is not growing. During this phase the hair falls out easily with combing or washing. About 13 percent of follicles are in the telogen phase at any one time, which accounts for the fact that the average person loses 70 to 120 hairs per day, depending on the amount of trauma to the scalp on any given day. Hair follicles rotate production similar to farmers rotating field crops. Some are dormant, but the rotating production of hair never shows because dormant follicles are dispersed over the entire scalp. All follicles and hair shafts are in different stages at any one time. If all the follicles were in the telogen phase at one time, there would be periods of total baldness, alternating with periods of thick growth throughout life. We see this phenomenon graphically when an animal sheds its hair.

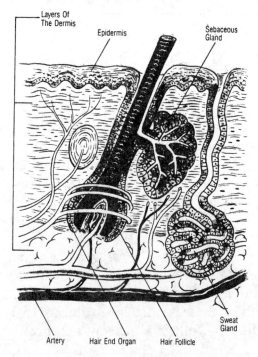

This is a normal hair in its follicle.

After the resting stage, a new growth cycle starts. This is the normal way in which healthy hair grows. When pattern baldness sets in, hair follicles begin to atrophy and hairs are not regrown.

Circulation Theory

One theory regarding baldness is that it is caused by too little blood circulation in the scalp. This theory has resulted in the creation of various remedies for the improvement of circulation. Some medical and non-medical practitioners give oral nicotinic acid to dilate scalp blood vessels. Massage is advocated by beauty salons and other non-medical clinics as a method of stimulating circulation, but although it imparts a pleasurable relaxing sensation, there is no reason to believe that it encourages hair growth. In fact, too much rubbing or pulling can induce hair loss. Heat treatments to increase scalp circulation and hence hair growth have been proposed, but this method has no foundation in fact.

There is nothing to indicate that poor circulation by itself is the cause of baldness. When hair follicles are transplanted into a bald area of the scalp, they flourish. This would not be possible if the cause of the baldness were inadequate circulation.

Another theory proposed is that an overabundance of circulation in the scalp causes baldness. This has given rise to the development of remedies to decrease the blood supply. Since normal levels of male hormone in the blood cause hair loss in susceptible individuals, researchers thought that reducing the exposure of the follicles to harmful hormones would reduce hair loss. Some surgeons experimented by tying off blood vessels to prevent circulation. This had no effect on the progression of baldness.

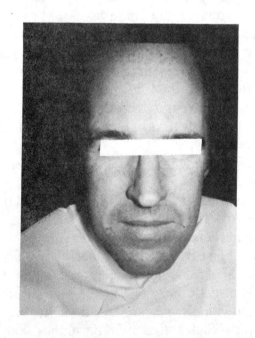

"U" shaped male pattern baldness.

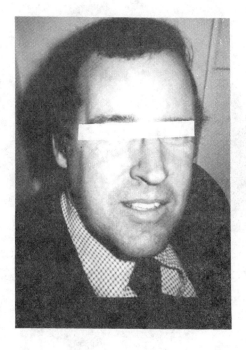

This type of baldness can be corrected by scalp reduction and hair transplantation.

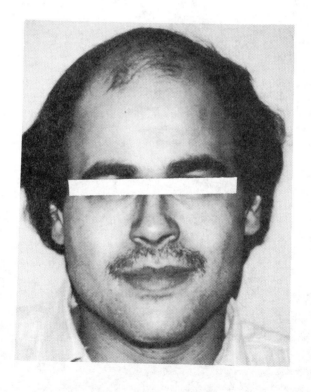

"U" shaped male pattern baldness.

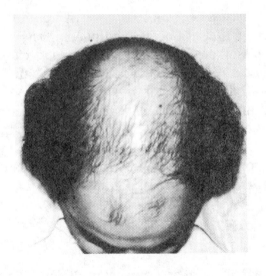

"U" shaped male pattern baldness.

Scalp Tightness Theory

Some researchers thought after studying the galea, the deep fibrous layer of scalp just above the skull, that if the galea were too tight, it could cause a restriction of scalp movement and result in hair loss. Some went so far as to make cuts through the skin to the galea in an effort to "loosen the scalp," but to no avail. One medical doctor in the Sunbelt region of America is currently studying galea thickness changes induced by ultrasonic devices, that he claims will induce hair re-growth.

Nutrition Theory

Although diet has been mentioned as one cause of male pattern hair loss, there is no evidence for such a claim. Certainly a proper diet contributes to good healthy hair. In extreme malnutrition, for example, or where there appears to be low levels of vitamin B, some temporary hair loss may occur. Extreme and chronic overdosage with vitamin A may result in temporary hair loss as well. Medical findings indicate that nutritional supplements will not reverse hair loss or stimulate hair re-growth in male pattern baldness.

Medical and Drug Theories

Although medical and surgical health problems may result in hair loss, none of these has been shown to contribute directly to male pattern loss. The role of stress may be important in the production of male hormones. This is still poorly understood as a mechanism. Many drugs can cause hair loss, especially anti-cancer agents.

Adjustment to Baldness

No discussion of the subject would be complete without touching on the alternative of accepting baldness as a natural human condition. This brings into play multiple psychological coping mechanisms which do work for many people. This is a normal, healthy way to adjust to imperfect situations. The assumption is made, however, that you are interested enough in alternatives to baldness to have read this far on the subject. No doubt you want to find ways of eliminating the less than acceptable fact of baldness.

Types of Baldness

There are varying degrees of baldness, ranging from thinness at the hair line to total baldness over the entire top of the head. For the sake of simplicity, this book repeatedly refers to the four usual types of baldness in the Western culture. Most men with balding problems fall somewhere within the range of these four types.

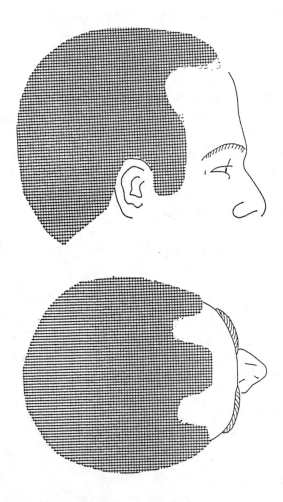

Type I. *This degree of baldness is depicted in the drawing as hair loss over the frontal area of the scalp up to 2 inches from where the average male had a normal hairline at age 12. It gives the appearance of a long, shiny forehead. Depending on the person's age, Type I baldness may progress no further or it may be the first stage of a progressive hair loss pattern. If the male is under 30 years of age, this type of baldness will most likely continue across the top of the scalp.*

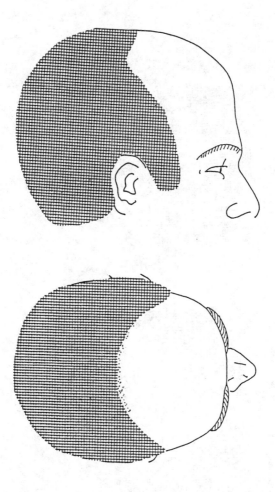

Type II. *This baldness extends to the top of the scalp from the normal hairline and is a common form of baldness for men 30 and older. It may be that the baldness will progress no further. By the time a man is 30, if there is no thinning in the posterior regions of the scalp, experience has shown that a person will rarely lose hair over the entire crown. Predictability of hair loss allows the doctor to recommend the best hair replacement approach for a 30-year-old or older patient.*

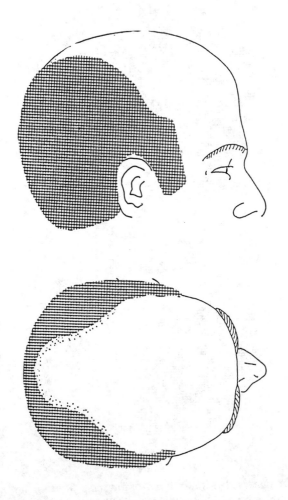

Type III. *This is the classic hair loss of a mature male.*

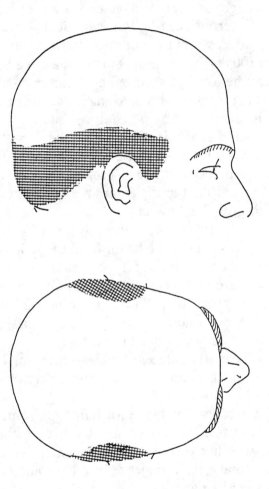

Type IV. *This type of baldness is the loss of hair from the frontal region deep into the posterior portion of the scalp. This leaves a fringe of hair circling the lower scalp. Usually there is an accompanying thinning of the remaining hair-bearing scalp along the sides of the head.*

Male pattern baldness depends on the interaction of androgens, age or time and genetics. As mentioned earlier, dihydrotestosterone, acting on genetically predisposed hair follicles, produces miniaturization of hair with resultant baldness. There are 100,000 hairs on the normal male scalp, but up to fifty percent can be lost before thinning is noticed—at least noticed by others. The person who is losing half of his hair is aware of it before it reaches a fifty percent loss.

The success of hair transplantation is based on transplanted hair follicles that will behave (grow) as they did in their original habitat and continue to grow in their new location. The secret is to transplant grafts from an area of the head that will continue to grow healthy hair.

For true Type I baldness, a series of grafts works well. Not many grafts need to be taken from the hair-bearing area to adequately cover the area of Type I baldness.

The male patient with Type II baldness may be a good candidate for grafts or a flap, depending on expectation and attitude. The remainder of the bald scalp can be adequately covered with a series of punch grafts.

The Type III baldness of males with high, ringed baldness may benefit from scalp reduction and numerous punch grafts (300 to 500).

The greatest challenge for hair replacement is Type IV baldness. Due to a wide need for donor hair, the doctor must determine whether or not hair replacement is possible. Once again, the final result depends on the quality of hair and motivation of the patient.

As with any classification, there are exceptions. Male pattern baldness can take any form, from baldness at the front or baldness on the crown of the scalp, to thin hair throughout or a combination. The doctor will be able to determine what results can best be achieved for a given hair problem. The following are a series of patterned hair loss examples that fall between the brackets of the classic four.

Patterned Hair Loss

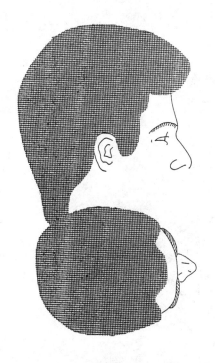

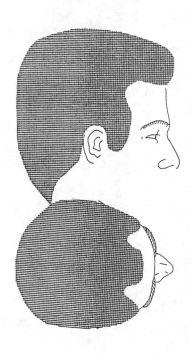

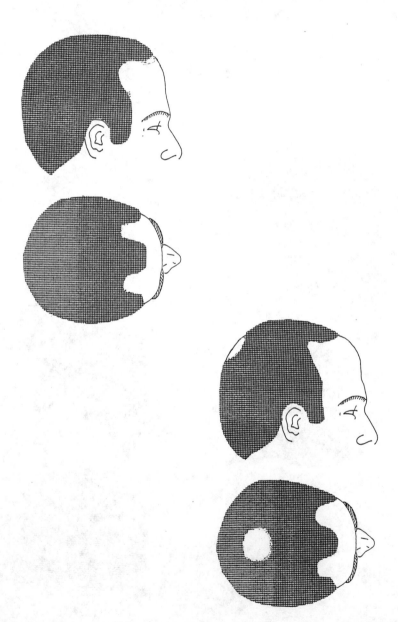

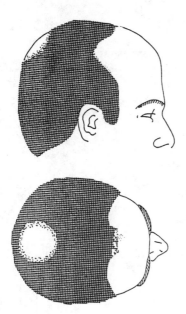

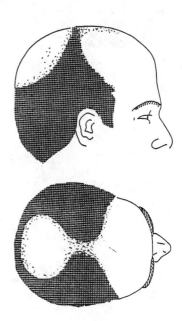

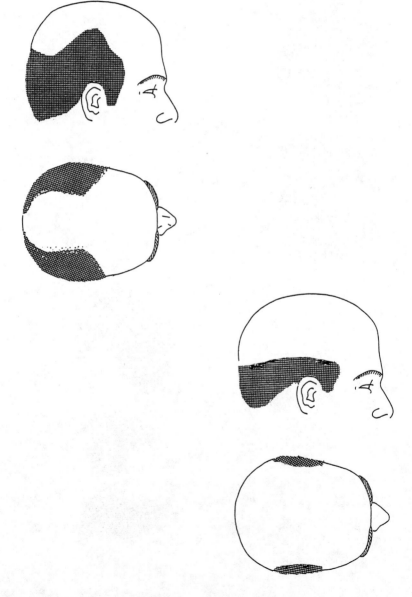

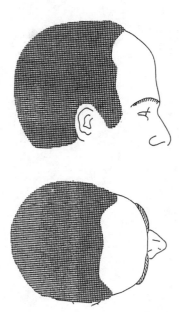

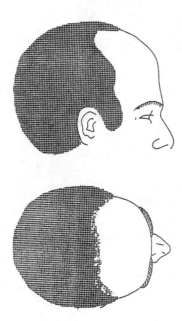

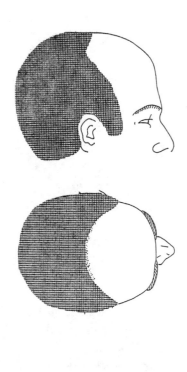

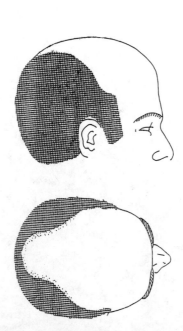

Chapter Four
Drugs, Hair and Treatment of Baldness

Various drugs are known to cause hair loss (notably the chemotherapeutic agents used in treating cancer), but none have been known to grow hair satisfactorily. Over a billion dollars a year is spent on hair growth remedies that include potions and drugs of every description. Those of us who are bald like to think that with current advanced technology there is some type of medication that will trigger hair growth.

Such drugs as Biotin have been advertised as a means to grow hair. Many advertisements make extravagant claims, but there has not been a scientifically proven case in which it has been effective. This also applies to over-the-counter products. Many of these potions are mail-order products that are not effective.

There have been dramatic statements about a new prescription drug that grows hair on the heads of some persons. The name of the new drug is minoxidil. It has been historically used in the treatment of high blood pressure. Today it is considered a remedy of last resort for hypertension due to its side effects. It was originally taken orally, and doctors noticed that some patients grew hair, often in unwanted areas of the body—the forehead or chest of women. This caused interest in its possible application to baldness and research has escalated in the past several years. Research has centered on the theory that as hair loss occurs, many of the hair follicles remain intact, thus allowing the possibility of re-growth. Of course, some follicles are atrophied or no longer productive, yet those present may be reactivated with use of minoxidil.

The drug minoxidil is dissolved in a liquid with alcohol as a base and applied to the scalp. Reports say five to twenty percent of patients applying the drug noted increased hair growth. When questioned about the quality of hair growth, it became clear that it was usually sparse—more like peach fuzz or down than normal hair. The more proper term is Vellus hair. Minoxidil is most useful in retarding hair loss. Though it has been approved for sale, research on minoxidil is still in its infancy and it remains to be seen what the results will be over an extended period of time.

Minoxidil, as a hair-restorer, has yet another drawback and that is the serious commitment to daily application. Once application of the expensive drug is discontinued, the new, fuzz-like hair that has grown will fall out. If a man in his twenties or thirties starts rubbing minoxidil into his scalp daily, he must commit to a regimen for life. It requires application twice a day and costs between $50 and $75 per month.

Experimental work has also been done with progesterone lotion and liquid injections into the scalp. The rationale is that progesterone competes with the chemical enzyme in the scalp to prevent the male hormone testosterone from breaking down into dihydrotestosterone which inhibits hair growth. If less dihydrotestosterone is formed from testosterone, there will supposedly be less hair loss. Reports suggest that progesterone injections have helped in some cases, but in general have limited effectiveness.

Researchers are also investigating a dozen other chemicals including hormones, all of which require extensive testing before government approval.

Beware of drugs and potions purporting to restore hair. At present, surgical treatment is the only truly successful medical aid for baldness.

Chapter Five

Hair Pieces and Fiber Implants

One surgical technique, that of implanting artificial hair fibers in the scalp, was a dismal, and in some cases disastrous failure. Implants should not be confused with transplants. Transplanting punch grafts is a useful and responsible surgical technique which has successfully corrected baldness in many people. Implants are done by surgically inserting synthetic fibers into the scalp with a needle. It was often performed by a non-medical person. For a time this technique was in vogue. Good quality fibers created an illusion of a full head of hair. Problems arose immediately. The implanted hair fibers broke off and caused infection. Some patients eventually had to have portions of their scalp removed because it was impossible to remove all the fibers that had broken off under the skin. The problem of infection was so extensive that governments passed laws prohibiting foreign body implants.

Hairpieces

Hairpieces provide a reasonable alternative to treating baldness. There is probably nothing easier or faster to apply. Hairpieces can be custom made in a short time and they look like a full head of hair. The drawbacks are that they can be easily detected and can be expensive and time-consuming to maintain.

The fibers in a hairpiece can be synthetic or human hair. Synthetic fibers last longer and are less expensive than human hair. They are not subject to discoloration due to sun exposure as is human hair. Human hair is far more expensive and doesn't last as long as synthetics, but it usually produces a more natural appearance. The use of hairpieces expanded rapidly, then leveled off.

Problems With Hairpieces

John Wayne wore a small hairpiece that seemed to please him, though he could have benefitted greatly from a hair transplant. At times he seemed weary of wearing it and was photographed in public without it. He learned, as have others, that a hairpiece is difficult to attach securely to the scalp.

One technique used to attach a hairpiece is called hair weaving. The wearer's existing hair is woven into the mesh base of the hairpiece to hold it in place. This secures the hairpiece quite effectively and causes the wearer less concern about having it dislodged. There is a disadvantage. The scalp under the mesh cannot be reached during normal cleansing, and skin secretions collect under the hairpiece. Even with daily shampooing, oil and scalp-flaking can collect, causing an unpleasant odor and even scalp problems. As the natural hair grows, the hairpiece becomes loose and must be reattached—about every six weeks. Re-weaving can cost from $60 to $80 each time it is done. Some hair breakage and hair loss can occur when the remaining hair is pulled or manipulated over a period of time.

Another technique to hold a hairpiece on the head is to attach it to sutures placed in the scalp. Stitches, usually coated wire, are inserted in the scalp and the base of the hairpiece is attached to them. This method is very reliable, but inadvisable since it can easily be a source of infection due to communication along the suture placements between the external environment and the underlying skin. Another disadvantage is that the wearer can't remove the hairpiece without stitches showing in the scalp. Should he ever decide to revert to his natural baldness, scars may be noticeable in the bald skin. This method of hair replacement was briefly popular, but it is performed less frequently now due to complications.

Hairpieces can also be affixed with adhesives placed on the bald skin; the hairpiece is applied with pressure and held in place for several seconds. Once the adhesive is set, the wearer can participate in normal activities. Still, there is always the fear of the hairpiece coming loose. For this reason surgeons developed the human skin loop to attach the hairpiece. For the human skin loop, the surgeon removes 2 to 3 cm of healthy skin from the abdomen and rolls the skin inside out to make a cylinder that is sutured together. The surgeon then makes an incision in the bald area of the scalp and sutures the cylinder to the scalp. It is much like a belt loop made of live human skin. A wire is placed through the cylinder of skin and is attached to the hairpiece. Once again, should the wearer tire of wearing a hairpiece, the cylinders remain permanently or until surgery is performed, which leaves unusual scaring.

The greatest disadvantage to wearing a hairpiece is psychological—fear of discovery. There is an ever-present sense of feeling false or that the hairpiece is not a part of the person.

An additional disadvantage is expense. Most quality hairpieces range form $1,000 to $3,000. Men generally require two hairpieces. One is a back-up to wear while the other is being cleaned and set or in case of damage to one. Most men prefer not to wear a hairpiece. They seek some other alternative.

An effective chemical treatment for baldness is yet to come. The hairpiece will always remain available and a good choice for some. But at present the most effective method to restore hair is surgical treatment using the patient's own hair as the source of replenishment of the bald area.

Chapter Six
Surgical Hair Replacement

Surgical methods to replace hair provide permanent results. This is true when hair is taken from the patient's own scalp in areas where he would never lose hair. Human hair, properly harvested, can be taken from any area of the body and grafted into most other parts of the body. Hair can be extracted from the side of the head and placed into the back of the hand or end of the nose and, properly grafted, will grow. It will grow as long as it was harvested from hair not programmed through heredity to fall out.

The current method of hair replacement by multiple punch autografts was described by Orentreich in 1959. Since then, the technique has undergone considerable refinement improving the cosmetic and therapeutic benefits. Hair transplantation is the most common operation performed on males today. It is estimated that more than one million bald patients have elected this procedure. Needless to say, there are many variations of hair grafts, but in the end, the result speaks for itself. A good hair transplant is not noticed as it usually goes undetected, but a poor result is always apparent.

Sophisticated techniques enable doctors to grow hair permanently on bald areas. Hair looks and grows exactly like the hair from the harvest site where it was removed. Precautions are taken in the transplantation procedure to ensure that hair growth direction is consistent.

Hair surgeons have developed variations on punch grafting to include hair strips and hair flaps.

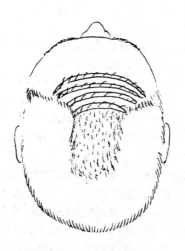

Example of strip grafting.

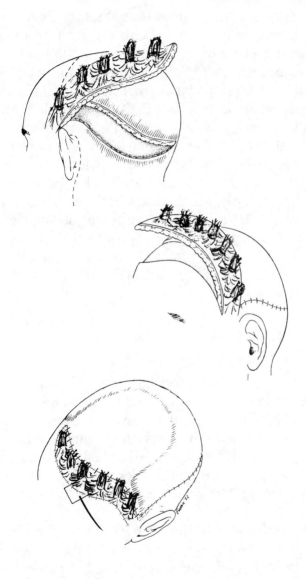

Example of Juri flap.

The strip was developed to allow for greater hair replacement with each strip, rather than the slower method of punch grafts. The greatest drawback to the strip procedures, besides the layering effect of strips across the scalp is adequate nourishment from surrounding blood supply in the scalp.

The flap was developed as a correction for male pattern baldness and its modified types of TPO flaps are designed to reach across the frontal scalp in a natural fashion. They give the patient considerably more peace of mind than previous methods.

There have been developmental problems, though. As mentioned, one disadvantage of the Juri flap has been that the flap hair grows posteriorly, which means in the wrong direction. In some patients, this has caused frustration with styling the hair. Today, men who have the flap are encouraged to have some form of hair control or permanent wave to change the direction of the hair. It is also a rather formidable surgical method that requires special surgical skill.

Punch Grafting

At present, the most popular form of surgical hair replacement is the punch grafting technique. In 1939, a Japanese surgeon, named Okuda, described the technique of punch grafting which he used in reconstruction of scarred scalps and eyebrows and pubic hair. He developed a method of removing small amounts of healthy hair on the sides and back of the head and then transplanting it to those areas where there was hair loss.

Due to World War II, his work went unnoticed by the world. Then in the 1950s, Dr. Norman Orentreich, a noted dermatologist in New York, unaware of Okuda's earlier work, experimented with hair replacement through punch grafting and reported his findings in medical journals. Since that time, the punch graft technique has grown in medical acceptance. When medical doctors applied the procedure to male pattern baldness, the hair replacement procedure took on greater meaning and spread rapidly.

The basic concept of punch grafting has been altered little since its introduction, though skilled physicians have improved on the technique and used innovative ways to make the hair transplants more natural looking. In addition to standard punch grafts, micro and mini grafts are used to create a more natural hairline. New instrumentation has also made the procedure much improved. It is basically a simple procedure in the hands of a well-qualified medical doctor.

The technique requires the doctor to surgically remove small circular pieces of hair-bearing skin—4 mm in diameter, from the back and sides of the head, and move these small grafts to the bald area of the scalp. The small spaces in the area from which the grafts were taken are either sutured together or left open to contract on their own and small, unnoticeable scars remain hidden by the surrounding hair that grows in a vertical or downward direction. There is rarely a visible cosmetic problem as long as the donor area is not too heavily harvested.

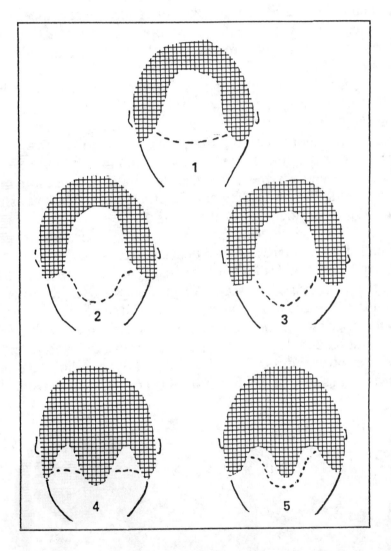

These illustrations show examples of proper and improper hairline placement. The most common error is shown in 4, while 1 is also undesirable, being too flat. Numbers 3 and 5 are the most desirable, if they are possible. Number 2, with a slight "flare" at each end, is acceptable (source: Norwood, 1984, p. 51).

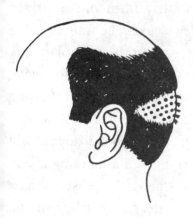

Donor area of grafts is at the back of the head.

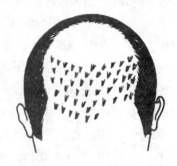

The donor hair from the back of the head has been grafted into the top of the head.

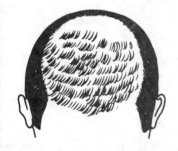

There is a period of time required for the grafts to reach styling length.

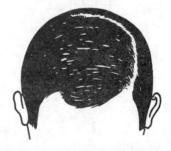

Months later the punch grafts have reached a length of growth that can be easily styled.

Most often, punch grafting is performed in the physician's office and done under local anesthesia. Following surgery, the patient merely requires an overnight dressing. After the transplants are completed, small scabs or crusts form on the surface of the grafts remaining for about three weeks. The trauma of the grafts being moved from the harvest site to the transplant site often causes the hair to fall out of the grafts four weeks following surgery. This condition is temporary. Three months following surgery, the transplanted hair follicles begin to grow hair again.

At the start of hair grafting, the medical doctor will outline the configuration of the hairline with a marking agent. This line will be symmetrical and an aesthetically pleasing shape. The patient is consulted on just where the new hairline should be, but it must be conservative and not placed too low on the forehead. It must fit the patient for life.

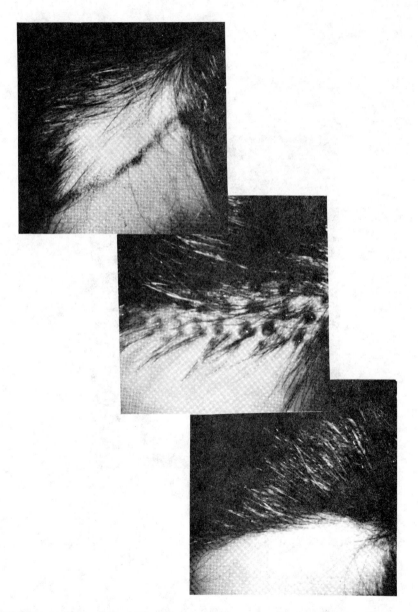

(1) The marking of the scalp; (2) the classic grafts; (3) the finished effect.

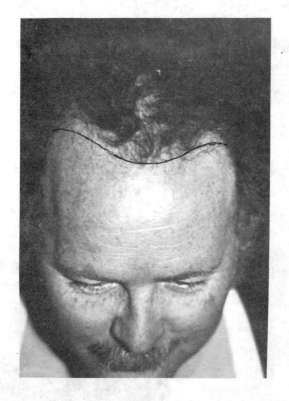

Before: This example shows the area the surgeon planned to graft, which has been marked with a line.

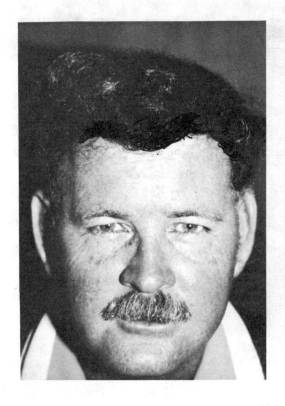

After: The desired effect was achieved in four sessions of grafting.

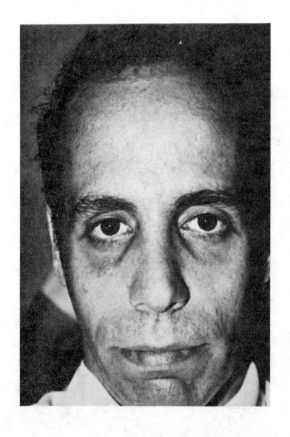

Before: The classic high forehead with male pattern baldness.

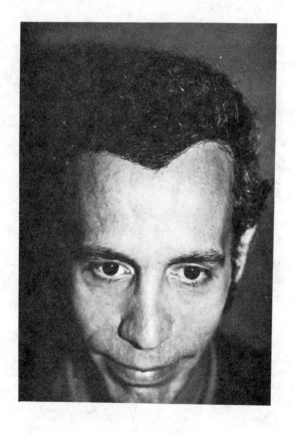

After: This man appeared ten years younger after hair transplantation.

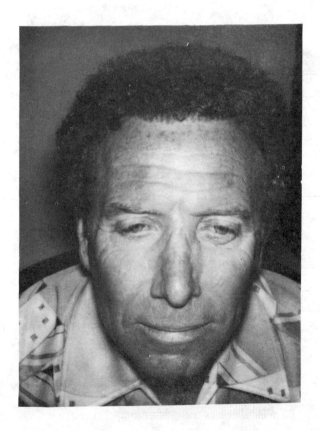

During Transplantation. Notice the grafts in the upper right of the frontal area.

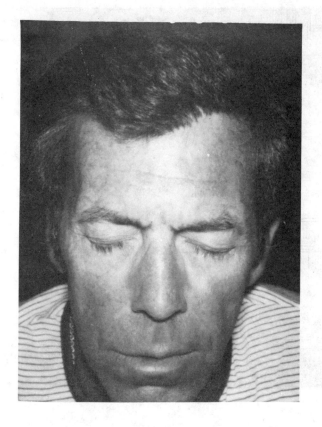

After: This man felt he had achieved a splendid result.

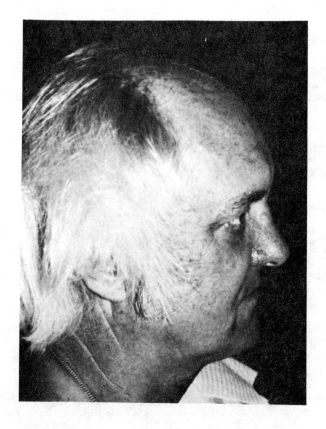

Before: This 57 year-old man had normal hair growth at the back of his head, but wanted a full styled appearance.

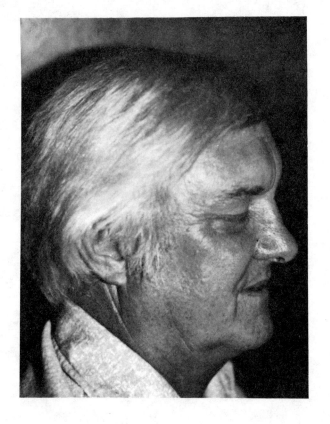

After: The frontal area of his hair was still sparse, but with proper styling, the result was pleasing.

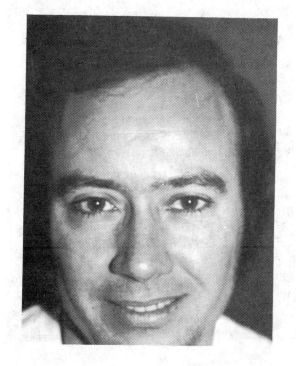

Before: This 31 year-old man wanted a more fully framed face.

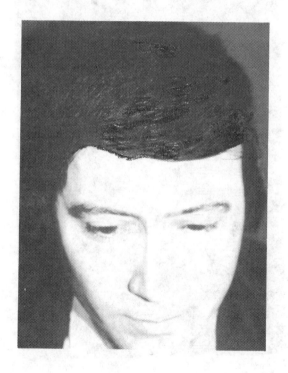

After: He achieved the full framing that gave him satisfaction.

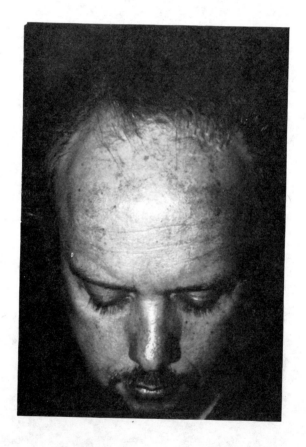

Before: This 42 year-old man had curly hair at the back of his head to use for grafts.

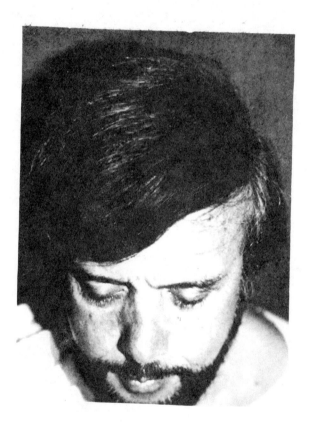

After: The grafts are also curly, and give him a full brushed look that is pleasing.

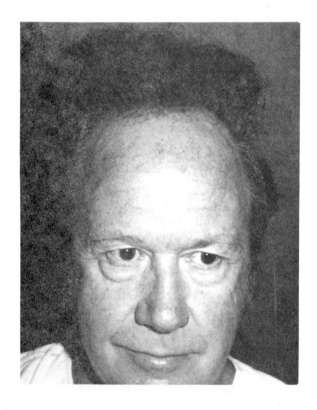

Before: This 48 year-old man had excellent coverage except for the classic frontal baldness.

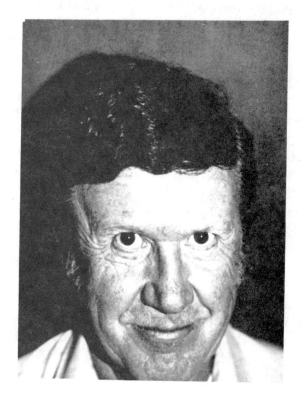

After: He is able to style his hair, much as he did 20 years earlier, after grafts were taken from the back of his head.

Most patients prefer a sharp angle at the juncture of the frontal and lateral hairline instead of a gradual gulf. These designs change as fashion and style dictate. Often the configuration of the frontal hairline dates the procedure. Many patients once requested a widow's peak, but medical records indicate that many patients now want a broad curved hairline.

The doctor will perform punch grafting in stages. That is, the first stage will establish a line by grafting as many as 50-60 grafts in three of four rows along the hairline. In the following sessions the doctor will place the grafts in a pattern that seems best for the full-hair look.

After a pause of about twelve weeks, the hair in the grafts begins to grow at the rate of half an inch a month, so that within eight months postoperatively, there will be hair growth of approximately two and a half inches in length.

It takes several sessions in the doctor's office to produce beneficial results. The grafts are placed one graft width apart to allow for adequate circulation. Grafts that do not receive an adequate blood supply will not survive or if they do survive they may yield few hairs. In subsequent sessions, the empty spaces are filled.

It takes approximately six months to complete four sessions. Each session requires from two to three hours, depending on the number of grafts to be implanted. Some patients need additional sessions to refine the final result. Most patients agree that the results are well worth the investment of time and money. Patients begin to see a realistic result after the first two sessions.

Pain

There is minimal pain with most punch autograf procedures. There may be some soreness or minor discomfor immediately following surgery. This discomfort can be alleviated with mild or moderate pain relievers. There may be minimal discomfort as well in the donor area for a week or two, especially if pressure is applied to the area.

Grooming

After surgery, the patient's activities are restricted for a week. Most can continue to work the next day. For the first week, the hair is washed carefully with a mild shampoo and groomed daily. As soon as the grafts are firmly established, the patient can resume normal activity.

Cost

The cost of hair transplants varies from doctor to doctor. It differs widely in various parts of the country. The price per graft ranges from $25 to $50. It is not unusual for a patient with moderate baldness to require 300 to 500 grafts.

Complications

Though serious complications are rare in punch grafts, certain problems may arise. If the hair follicles are injured at the time of surgery, or if too many grafts are performed at one time, some of the follicles may be lost due to lack of proper blood circulation in the growth area. An experienced medical doctor avoids complications.

Patients seeking hair-replacement surgery are concerned about scarring. Whenever the scalp is incised, some scarring occurs. If the grafts grow well, however, little scarring is apparent. The scars tend to be hidden by overlying hair.

Hundreds of thousands of men have had successful punch grafts and have enjoyed years of fuller hair. It is one of the most proven methods of hair restoration available and is the most frequent operation performed on males today.

Chapter Seven
Scalp Reduction

Scalp reduction is another remedy for baldness and is commonly done to aid punch grafting. If the bald area is reduced in size, then the remaining bald skin requires fewer grafts to fill. Scalp reduction is a technique that involves bringing the dense permanent side hair closer to the crown thereby reducing the size of the bald spot. Scalp reductions have been performed successfully for seventy-five years, though mainly in conjunction with removal of tumors or scars on the scalp. The application of this procedure as a remedy for baldness has evolved only in the last decade and has become an important part of hair replacement surgery.

The Scalp Reduction Process

Scalp reduction means that a part of the bald scalp is cut out or excised. The surrounding skin and hair are then stretched upward tightly to pull the thicker hair from the sides toward the top of the scalp. The scalp, in most cases, is mobile and lax. Scalp reduction is most often performed in conjunction with the procedure of punch grafts. It is effective and safe. A reduction allows the surgeon to place more needed grafts in the frontal area of the scalp.

When part of the bald scalp is removed and the incision closed, the scalp feels tight. The patient is aware of the tightness for several days.

Scalp reduction can be repeated, further reducing the size of the bald area. These procedures can be done four to eight weeks apart. Scalp reduction is an office procedure and discomfort usually lasts a short period of time. The day after surgery the patient rarely experiences any pain, though there may be some tenderness to the touch for a few days.

One major advantage to scalp reduction surgery is that it doesn't require a significant interruption of the patient's personal or professional life. If a patient is from out of town, he can travel to the doctor's office, have the reduction performed and return to the surgeon's office the next morning, have his bandage removed and return home. He will look much better than when he entered the doctor's office.

Should the patient be from out of the area, a medical doctor or an assistant in the patient's home area can usually remove the staples two weeks following surgery. The staples are not visible if the patient has a reasonable amount of hair. If they are visible then a cap can be worn or a strip bandage placed over the stapled area of the scalp.

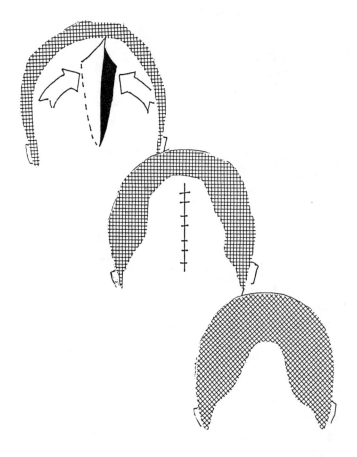

These illustrations show how scalp reduction works. First an incision is made and the scalp is pulled toward the bald area on top. Excess skin is cut away and the scalp is sewn together. This may be carried out several times, depending on the need of the individual and the flexibility of his scalp. Finally, the bald area that remains can be implanted with plugs taken from the sides and back.

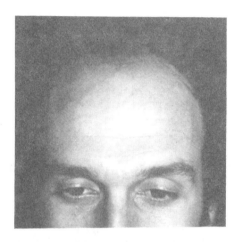

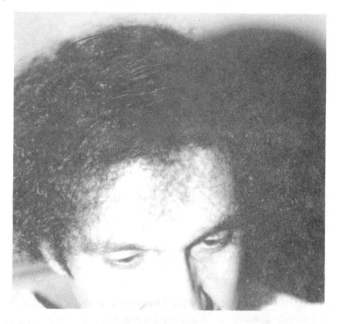

The results after scalp reduction and punch grafting.

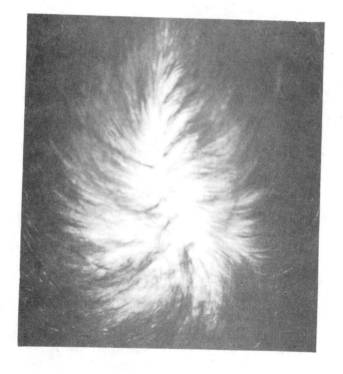

Grafts are placed into scalp reduction scar and grow very well.

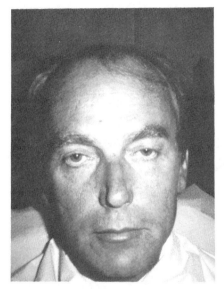

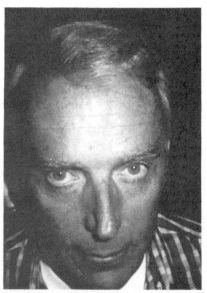

After scalp reduction, punch grafting and mini-grafting give a more natural appearance.

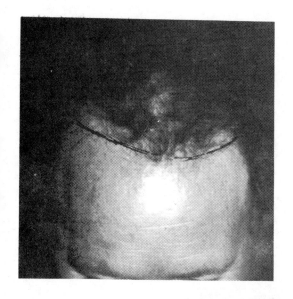

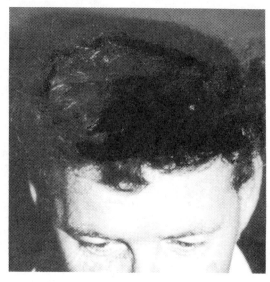

The final result after punch grafts and mini and micro grafts. The area is replenished with a full head of hair.

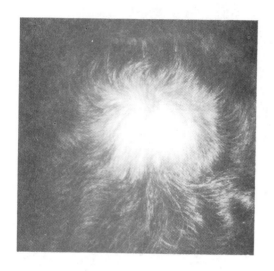

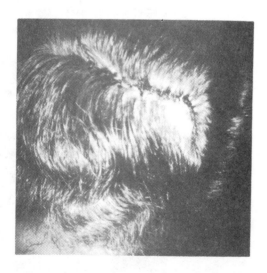

A scalp reduction immediately post-operative (staples in place.)

Chapter Eight

Patient Selection and Hair

The Medical Examination

Before scheduling for a transplantation, consultation is essential. You as the patient will be carefully evaluated and the procedure explained in detail so that you will understand what is involved. For the doctor to perform hair transplants you must be able to tolerate local anesthesia. Most patients with baldness are in such good physical condition as to obviate concern for anesthesia. Should there be a question, the possible existence of an underlying disease which might constitute a surgical risk, must be determined.

Scalp Condition

The hair replacement surgeon will examine the scalp to determine any dermatological problems that could interfere with surgery. Sores, open wounds or rash may need to be corrected before transplants are started. Dandruff, which is known as seborrheic dermatitis, is not a contraindication to surgery, but the condition should be treated.

Donor Area

The hair density and quality of the donor area must be considered to determine if there is an adequate supply of healthy hair to harvest. The best candidates for hair transplantation have sufficient donor hair of adequate density. Age is not a determining factor, as long as you are in good health. Light or gray hair appears denser as there is less contrast between hair and scalp. Curly hair covers much better than straight hair because it appears thicker. This is why a permanent wave in the transplanted hair often improves appearance, as well as reduces the grooming time.

When To Transplant Hair

The question of when to start hair transplantation is difficult to answer. Many start when there is sufficient alopecia (pattern baldness) that can be corrected and before it is apparent that the patient has lost a great deal of hair. Thus, the healing wounds can be covered by the existing hair. It is also important to start hair transplantation while the patient is relatively young. Hair is important to a young person with an active social life and who is trying to forge ahead in the business community. At the other end of the spectrum, there are those in their 60s and 70s desirous of hair transplantation in which very good results have been a achieved and the feeling is one of a more youthful person.

Before surgery, laboratory studies are performed. These include a complete blood count, serum chemistry profile, coagulation studies, syphilis screen, hepatitis screens, and a test for acquired immunodeficiency syndrome. Patients who have abnormal laboratory studies must be evaluated medically before surgery.

Preoperatively patients are placed on vitamin K twice daily beginning 1 week before surgery. This reduces the incidence of bleeding and helps with coagulation. Before surgery, erythromycin (an antibiotic) is instituted twice daily and continued for 1 week post operatively. In addition, the patient receives an injection of cortisone at surgery. This is most important in reducing edema (fluid) and postoperative inflammation.

The surgeon considers the patient's wishes as to style of hair, design and shape whenever possible. The medical doctor will determine, if need be, how many scalp reductions the bald area may require. The reduction is usually performed as a longitudinal midline excision.

Age

If the patient is under 25 years of age it may be difficult to predict the final extent of eventual baldness. Family history will provide the doctor with some indication. If the patient is under 25 years of age the surgeon will probably take a conservative approach to correcting baldness. With experience the doctor can estimate future hair loss based on the patient's age, degree of baldness, and family history. Patients, 40 and over, may have an established pattern of baldness that is predictable.

Timing Treatment Periods

Patient and surgeon can work out a schedule for treatment periods, usually no closer than three or four weeks. If scalp reduction is needed, reductions are usually spaced about 4-8 weeks apart. Keep in mind that the entire process can take up to a year or more, depending on patient motivation, type of baldness and number of grafts required.

Photographs

Photographs are usually taken prior to the first session. In this manner the patient and surgeon can check progress. As happens with other cosmetic surgical procedures, there is a tendency to forget what the baldness was like prior to hair transplant surgery. It is surprising to see the dramatic change that occurs toward the end of the sessions.

Many experienced hair transplant surgeons are experts at correcting problems that may have been created by less experienced doctors or by patients themselves. There also are new innovative procedures in use today that were not available a few years ago. This allows patients, who previously had treatments, to return and take advantage of new developments in hair replacement.

Instrumentation

Hair surgeons now use the latest instruments to remove punch grafts from their original site. The original punches used for hair transplant surgery were hand-held, and the surgeon twisted and pushed or just pushed downward in cookie cutter fashion to cut the graft. One of the most significant advances in hair transplant surgery was the development of the power punch. Superior quality grafts and thus more hair growth are obtained, while at the same time enhancing patient comfort during the procedure. Obviously, patients prefer the power punch over the hand punch. It is essential that the punch instrument be exquisitely sharp or else the graft will be distorted. A sharp punch cuts without pressure, and the grafts are broader at the base than at the skin surface. Also it is important that the punch be sharp at the recipient site. This is the bald area of the scalp where skin must be removed to create a tight fitting, circular hole for the graft to be inserted.

Postoperative Care

An antibiotic ointment is placed over the grafts and donor site to ward off any potential infection. This then is covered with gauze and a pressure dressing. Spray adhesive is used on recipient sites by some surgeons in place of the pressure dressing. The dressing is left overnight and removed the following morning when the patient returns to the office. At this time the scalp is cleansed and the grafts checked to determine if any have become dislodged or turned in a wrong direction. A crust will form over each graft and remain for about 3 weeks. An interesting event happens about the fourth week when the hair in the grafts shed, then in 10 to 16 weeks after surgery, regrow.

Minigrafts and Micrografts

A problem that long existed with hair transplantation was the tendency to produce a hairline that was too abrupt and too thick. A natural hairline is not really a line but a transitional zone between the bald skin of the forehead and the thick, uniform density of the frontal forelock. Micro and minigrafts are used to soften the frontal hairline. This makes it less abrupt and reduces the tufted effect. Minigrafts, consisting of three or more hairs, are obtained by sectioning 4.5 mm grafts into halves and the halves into quarters. The minigraft is placed in the scalp after creating a slash would with a scalpel blade at a point slightly anterior to or between the spaces in the hairline. The wound heals without scarring and the hairs appear very natural.

A micrograft consists of one or two hairs and is obtained by teasing intact hairs from the periphery of the standard graft. A stab wound is made with a needle and the hair is threaded into the hole.

Micro and minigrafts are placed as close as possible to the first row of grafts and at the same angle to the skin. A slightly irregular placement mimics the normal irregularity of the natural hairline.

Complications

Hair transplantation complications are rare. Postoperative bleeding can occur but is not usual. Because the scalp is so vascular, infection is extremely uncommon, especially when prophylactic antibiotics are used. Postoperative edema (fluid) may occur when transplanting the frontal area of the scalp, especially following the first session. This can be diminished with the use of systemic corticosteroids. Pain in the postoperative period is minimal and responds to mild analgesics. Hypesthesia (numbness) can occur as a result of cutting peripheral nerve endings. Sensation usually returns in 2 to 3 months. Sparse growth and scarring are usually due to poor technique as is cobblestoning or elevation of the grafts. Revisions are possible with an experienced hair surgeon.

The art and science of hair transplantation has come a long way since its introduction. Both technique and instrumentation, as well as aesthetic considerations, have greatly improved, thus offering the patient a vastly superior cosmetic result that will last a lifetime.

Chapter Nine
Procedure

With a better understanding of the surgical procedure of hair transplantation and the advice on follow-up visits, it is essential to make contact with the medical doctor you have selected to perform the procedure. Remember that the doctor may want to take a history of what you have tried before. He may want you to have a physical examination. Most likely, before the end of the first visit you will learn whether or not you should have a hair transplant. The medical doctor, during the consultation, will explain costs and indicate when he can begin the procedure. During the consultation visit, be sure to ask questions and get the answers you need to proceed comfortably with the treatment.

The doctor will determine what is surgically correctable and just how much donor hair is available for hair replacement. He may evaluate the need for scalp reduction. The doctor may recommend a scalp reduction or perhaps a series of scalp reductions. Don't be alarmed. This has become standard procedure for many patients to obtain the maximum hair coverage for the bald area of the scalp. Scalp reduction pulls together the bald area.

The day of treatment you will be placed in a well-equipped outpatient room. You will probably be seated much like you have been in a dentist's chair and preparations will get underway to anesthetize the donor and recipient regions of the scalp. Once there is no feeling in these regions, healthy grafts will be removed from the donor area (most often at the back of the head) with a sterile instrument that makes a small round hole to obtain the graft.

Depending on the size of the graft needed, the doctor will remove plugs containing as many as 20 hairs per graft. Of course the density of the donor site will determine the number of hairs per graft. An average punch contains 10 to 15 hairs and is about 4 mm in diameter.

Procedure

The average frontal hairline is five to six rows deep and requires at least four sessions of 4-mm grafts placed into 3.5-mm recipient holes. This differential between graft and recipient site results in a close approximation as the graft tends to shrink when removed from the donor site, while the recipient site tends to expand. There are variations when a 0.25-mm differential or a 0.75-mm differential is required. To maintain adequate vascular supply, intact skin, 3.5 mm in diameter is left between each graft. The hair surgeon follows a pattern that allows adequate space between each graft during each session. Spaces should be left between each graft and an empty row between each row after the first session. In the second session, grafts fill the spaces between the first grafts; the third and fourth sessions will fill between the rows. It takes at least four sessions to approximate the grafts in any given area.

Grafts are placed at an acute angle of 20 to 30 degrees producing a shingled effect as the hair grows. Keeping the hair low to the scalp and growing forward results in a natural appearance and greater coverage.

Following removal of the donor grafts from the back of the head, the plug-like grafts are placed in a saline solution in a Petri dish. They are never allowed to dry out while they await insertion into the receptor site. After discarding skin from the recipient site, hemostasis is obtained, and the scalp is cleansed with hydrogen peroxide. The grafts are then inserted into the recipient site. Hairs are placed in an anterior direction, and the best grafts are put into the most strategic locations, usually anterior and on the part side.

What about the small holes left at the donor site on the back of the head? Most transplant surgeons do not routinely suture the donor site. Many feel that it they suture the holes, there will be a slight scalp reduction in reverse. In other words, the suturing may pull together the donor site, but in so doing it may stretch the bald area of the crown.

The doctor will transplant only a limited number of grafts at any one treatment session. The patient is asked to return for additional transplants at varying intervals. This allows the previous transplants time to heal.

Risks of hair transplant surgery are not the normal risks associated with general surgery. Transplants involve the skin only. This is why complications are rare. In any surgery there is the possibility of infection, but this too is rare. The doctor asks the patient to take precautions to keep the scalp clean and free from contamination.

It will take twelve weeks for the hair grafts to grow, but in time the transplants grow as vigorously as normal hair would on the back of the head. When the hair begins to grow, the patient may wish to visit a hair stylist who is experienced with hair grafts. This experienced person can give the hair a fuller appearance.

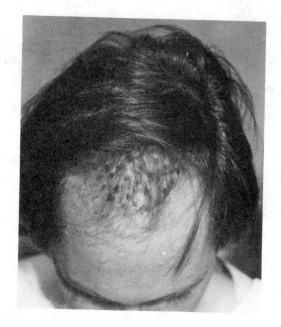

Normal Punch Grafts.

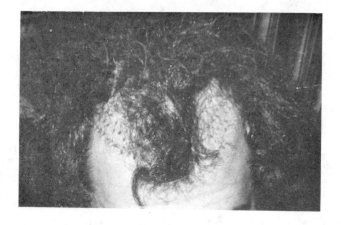

Mini punch grafts.

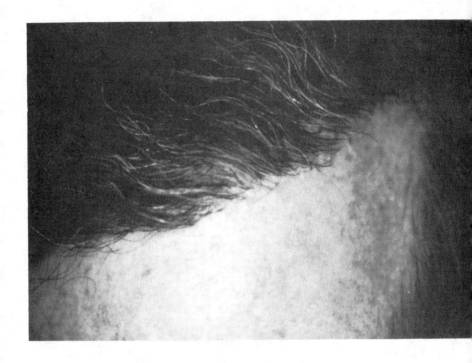

Micro punch grafts.

Bald Scalp Reduction

One of the most effective methods for reducing the number of punch grafts need to fill up a bald space is bald scalp reduction. If you take your hands and press them to sides of your head and push in and upward you may notice that your scalp is loose and flexible. If the scalp loose and you can see a wrinkling in the center of your bald spot, chances are you have excess bald scalp that can be excised in a pre-designed pattern to reduce the total bald area of your head.

Bald scalp reduction makes hair transplantation candidates out of patients who ordinarily would be too bald to achieve significant results. For patients with extensive baldness, conventional hair transplantation often will not be sufficient or satisfactory because donor sites are inadequate and cannot yield enough autografts to cover bald scalps effectively. If a large enough area of baldness is excised (surgically removed) from the scalp, the grafts may become sufficient, as it has been estimated that bald scalp reduction will save five to nine grafts per square centimeter of excised scalp.

Bald scalp reduction began in the late 1970s and has become a standard procedure when needed. Normally, the bald scalp can be removed and the hair-bearing part of the scalp pulled together in three or four sessions over a period of 6 months. Most scalps are fairly stretchable and even those that are not very elastic can be made more so by vigorous massage daily for several weeks. If the scalp remains too tight to be totally reduced, hair transplants can be placed in the remaining bald portion.

The scar resulting from bald scalp reduction usually is a fine surgical scar, but occasionally it tends to spread. In such cases, transplants can be placed into the scar itself with adequate growth.

Although the usual procedure is to do all the scalp reductions first and then follow with hair transplants, some patients prefer to alternate between scalp reductions and hair transplantation. Surgery can be done every 6 weeks, alternating scalp reduction and hair transplants. However, if the anterior hairline is transplanted prior to scalp reduction, the lateral portion may be pulled posterior and must later be corrected.

Postoperative

The medications and dressing for scalp reduction are much the same as with hair transplantation. The hair surgeon will apply antibiotic medication, dress the scalp with a Kling or Conform pressure dressing and have the patient return the following day.

Complications are rare. Headaches during the first 24 hours after surgery are not uncommon. It is important that the patient receives adequate pain medication to alleviate this problem.

Chapter Ten
Hair Transplant Questions

How successful are hair transplants?

In skilled hands they have proven most successful. Satisfaction depends to a great extent on the patient's expectations. The hair is "redistributed" in this procedure and the patient cannot expect hair as thick over the entire scalp as it was before baldness began.

How long will transplanted hair last?

Transplanted hair should LAST A LIFETIME, or at least as long as the hair remains in the region from which the transplants were harvested. This conclusion is based on examinations over the past 30 years showing continued growth of hair after the first transplants were performed.

Who should have hair transplants?

Baldness is not limited to any economic, social or ethnic group; neither is the desire for restoration of one's hair. Truck drivers, bankers, firemen, laborers and lawyers, men and women in all walks of life have received hair transplantation, making it a popular office surgical procedure.

What type of baldness makes this procedure helpful?

a.   Male Pattern Baldness, the most common form of hair recession in men.

b.   Baldness from scars resulting from burns, accidents, surgery or radiation.

c.   Baldness from infections, including ringworm, boils or folliculitis.

d.   Baldness from systemic disease, such as high fever, shock or nervous conditions.

e.   Absence of eyebrows.

What is the procedure?

The donor area at the back of the scalp is anesthetized, using local anesthesia. The number of grafts to be transplanted are then removed with a special power instrument. Next, the bald area is similarly anesthetized and small punch areas are removed and discarded. The transplants are specially cleaned and prepared, then carefully placed into the recipient sites. A temporary dressing is applied and this is removed the following day.

Is the procedure painful?

Most patients have said there is little or no pain involved. Those who have some mild discomfort and soreness find that they are readily relieved by mild analgesics.

How do most patients accept this procedure?

Acceptance by patients has been excellent, especially those who have previously pursued non-surgical methods of hair replacement. Nothing is so gratifying as seeing one's own hair growing where there had previously been none.

How many sessions does it take to achieve the final desired effect?

This varies with each patient. The average series of transplants sessions is four or five.

How long does each procedure take?

This varies with the number of transplants done, but normally will take about two hours.

What percentage of the transplants "take" or grow hair?

This depends on the experience and skill of the surgeon. Usually the only transplants lost have been due to patients inadvertently combing or "uprooting" the transplants before they had completely healed.

How long does it take hair transplants to grow?

The transplanted hair is usually shed in four weeks and about eight weeks later new hair begins to grow and continues to grow at the normal rate of 1/2 inch per month. Some patients do not shed the original transplants, but experience growth from the time of the transplantation. However, these are unusual cases.

How should a patient prepare himself for the procedure?

Patients are usually seen in consultation prior to any procedure. During this interview the patient has the opportunity to ask any questions. The patient is asked to complete a medical history and routine lab work is performed before starting a series of hair transplant sessions. Intake of analgesics, such as aspirin, should be restricted as they may cause bleeding. Alcoholic beverage intake should also be restricted just prior to and immediately following the procedure. The hair should be shampooed the night before and the day of the procedure.

Should you have a haircut prior to the procedure?

The hair should be left long so that it will cover areas of the scalp following surgery.

What can I do after immediately following treatment?

Most patients may resume their normal activities unless they involve strenuous physical activity. Bandages will remain in place until the next day. These are preferably removed in the doctor's office, at which time the hair is cleansed and each patient is given detailed, written instructions on the exact care of the transplants.

How much does it cost?

This varies with the individual and the extent of the hair loss, but generally speaking, the procedure is no more expensive than a good hairpiece, which would cover the same area. All fees will be thoroughly discussed at the time of the initial consultation.

Can I be put to sleep during the hair transplant procedure?

This has on rare occasions been done but most patients find that the office procedure has proven almost pain-free with a local anesthetic, less expensive, more convenient, and without the risk of complications that accompanies general anesthesia.

Are there any complications with the procedure?

This has been infrequent and only of minor concern. Bleeding is rarely a problem and is controlled with pressure. Infection is rare and medications are given in advance to offset any such problems. Some patients experience swelling, usually only after the first session.

Can I continue to wear a hairpiece during the growth of the hair transplants?

Yes. This often serves as a protective shield and an excellent cosmetic screen, so long as it is removed daily and the transplanted area is thoroughly cleaned. In extensive cases of baldness there may be inadequate donor hair to cover the entire area, and then transplanted hair may be used for a frontal hairline to enhance the natural appearance of the hairpiece.

Will there be any visible scars?

As with any cosmetic surgical procedure, if the patient is closely examined, extremely minimal, obscure scar lines can be detected.

What happens to the donor site from which the transplants are taken—will it be bald?

No. This is one of the most important features of the procedure. After the transplants are removed, the donor sites shrink to very small pinhead size scars and are well hidden by the surrounding hair that grows in a downward direction on the back of the head. Amazing as it may seem, more than 500 hair grafts have been taken from the back of the head without producing a visual cosmetic defect.

Overall, hair transplants have given satisfaction to hundreds of thousands of patients over the decades that it has been performed. No matter what your hair problem, you cannot outguess the medical doctor, experienced in the field of hair transplant treatments, as to whether or not you are a candidate. Let the doctor examine you and let him give an evaluation as to whether you can have the procedure. You may be overjoyed with the results of his evaluation and solution to your problem of baldness.

Sample Instructions
Preceding Hair Transplant Surgery

(The following are general instructions. Your surgeon may have other specific items that will be included in his instructions that are slightly different then these.)

1. Obtain the required blood tests at least three weeks prior to the transplant surgery. These tests must be done before eating breakfast.

2. Completely avoid aspirin (acetylsalicylic acid) at least one week prior to the procedure. Note this medication is contained in many common drugstore over-the-counter products, including Alka Seltzer, Bufferin, Excedrin, Empirin, Dristan, etc. You may take analgesics such as Tylenol or Valadol.

3. Do not drink alcoholic beverages for one week prior to surgery. If you wish a relaxant or tranquillizer, please request appropriate medication when you arrive at the office.

4. Use the prescribed medicated shampoo regularly. It is recommended that you shampoo the night before and the morning of the procedure. (You should continue to use this shampoo after the procedure, as directed.)

5. Do not shorten the hair on the back of the head (in the donor area) prior to the procedure.

6. Do not wear a pullover shirt on the day of your surgery.

7. Eat a light meal approximately one or two hours before coming to the office. Do not completely skip breakfast or lunch,

and do not eat a heavy meal immediately before the procedure. Maintain normal intake of food and liquids during the days preceding the surgery.

8. You should plan to return the next morning, at which time your head will be unwrapped and thoroughly cleaned. If you live a great distance, plan to remain in the area for a couple of days.

9. You will be given a complete written set of instructions following surgery.

10. Due to the fact that hair transplant procedures are usually booked one to three months in advance, give two weeks notice to cancel or change an appointment. If you give less notice and the doctor is unable to schedule another patient in your stead, you may forfeit your deposit.

11. The fee for transplant surgery is to be paid the day of the surgery, less the deposit.